OVERCOMING
DEPRESSION

OVERCOMING DEPRESSION

One Christian's Perspective

Marilyn Okoye

Marilyn Okoye

Unless otherwise noted, all Scripture quotations are taken from the King James Version (KJV) of the Holy Bible.

Scripture quotations marked AMP are taken from The Amplified® Bible, copyright © 1954, 1958, 1962, 1964, 1965, 1987 by The Lockman Foundation. Used by permission.

Scripture quotations marked MSG are taken from *The Message* by Eugene H. Peterson, copyright © 1993, 1994, 1995, 1996, 2000, 2001, 2002. Used by permission of NavPress Publishing Group. All rights reserved.

Scriptures of Encouragement and Affirmations excerpts taken from "Who You Are In Christ". Used by permission. *www.concernedchristians.com*

To contact the author for book signings or speaking engagements, please send email to: overcomingdepression@livingwatercreations.com

Edited by Jason N. Robinson

Forewords by
Pastor Beverly L. Wilson
and Mildred L. Heath

Make-up by Adriane Anderson

Photos by TS Design Studio

This book was printed in the United States of America.

To order additional copies of this book, contact:
Xlibris Corporation
1-888-795-4274
www.Xlibris.com
Orders@Xlibris.com
28496

Dedication

This book is dedicated to my mom. Many years ago I saw your pain. I did not comprehend its depth; however, I knew it was there, and I knew it was deep. After that, I saw your strength. I did not understand its magnitude; nevertheless, you bore the weight of your struggle while you held our family together. Finally, I witnessed your determination. I tried to ascertain its value; overtime, it became the example I chose to follow, the invaluable principle that kept me focused. Mom, you have given me a foundation of love, hope, and faith, established on the Word of God. Thank you for training me in the way I should go.

To my children, Jazzmin, Emmanuel, Jr., and Amalachukwu—lessons lived are lessons learned; lessons missed are lessons that will have to be repeated. It's okay to learn something from someone else's lessons. Pain, strength and determination, love, hope and faith—they are all a part of life's lessons; don't miss them.

To my siblings, Robert, Maurice, Latrecha, Ericka, Michelle, and Christopher, my family and extended family both here and afar—the sky's the limit, let the Holy Spirit be your guide.

This book is also dedicated to the sweet memories of my dad, Melvin L. Sandifer.

CONTENTS

PRAYERS OF ENCOURAGEMENT
AND AFFIRMATIONS

SCRIPTURES OF ENCOURAGEMENT
AND AFFIRMATIONS

Acknowledgements

God Almighty, I have seen You as the "I am that I am."

Special Thanks:

To Margaret Latham: God's grace has been exemplified in your compassion toward me. I thank God that you believed in me, for me and with me. Although I don't fully comprehend God's grace toward me, I do comprehend that our lives intersected so that the Holy Spirit would illuminate a part of its (grace's) understanding to me. Thank you for your kindness, understanding, support, and encouragement.

To Mildred L. Heath: You were a surrogate mom to me. Your words were full of wisdom and truth. For that, I am eternally grateful to God that He had planned our meeting even before we were born.

To RMC: I've only known you for a short period of time, but I am so happy our paths have crossed. There is a calm that exists within you that we should all aspire to have. Thank you for your light!

To Audrey: Words cannot express the gratitude I have in my heart toward you. Over 27 years ago, you became a special part of my life that I know many may never understand. But it is so good to know that our thoughts are not His thoughts and that our ways are not His ways.

I am grateful for all spiritual leaders in my life, past and present. Apostle H. Daniel Wilson and Pastor Beverly L. Wilson, my spiritual parents since 1993, have helped to equip me for the work of God's Kingdom. Thank You! To a host of supporters, far too many to name, I thank God for all of your words of comfort and encouragement. To a special group of women whom I love dearly, thank you for sharing my pain: Eugenia Brown, Amanda Anderson, Sandra Caldwell, Cynthia Baldwin, Dr. Sharon Dominguez, Andrea Martin, Andrea Williams, and Gloria Johnson. To Angela, Darla, Natalie, Tonya, and my entire VKMI family—Love ya!

To Jason N. Robinson: Thank you for your time and your grammatical expertise. This has been a learning experience that I will treasure for the rest of my life. As you diligently probed each page of this book, your editorial passion and keen eyesight for every oversight were invaluable tools that God used to help shape this book into its divine purpose.

Foreword

Do you open your eyes in the morning and feel like you want to close them again and just sleep all day? Do you feel that you've disappointed not only those loved ones in your life but also yourself? Do you sometimes feel helpless, hopeless, and bitter about your current life circumstances? Well, . . . Guess What, . . . THAT'S NORMAL!! Emotional feelings are a natural part of our fleshly body. It is possible for you to feel down and depressed as if your life has no meaning at all. But, there is a cure for being free from this emotional roller coaster.

Even if you have to take prescription medicine for a season, the good news is you don't have to depend on it for the rest of your life. The ultimate cure is from the Creator of all living flesh, our Heavenly Father, God. God's word is our daily prescription, and it is the ultimate cure for any of life's situations.

✝ Phil. 1:6—"And I am sure that God who began the good work within you will keep right on helping you grow in his grace until his task within you is finally finished on that day when Jesus Christ returns."

✝ Phil. 4:6-7—"Don't worry about anything; instead, pray about everything; tell God your needs and don't forget to thank him for his answers. If you do this you will experience God's peace, which is far more wonderful than the human mind can understand. His peace will keep your thoughts and your hearts quiet and at rest as you trust in Christ Jesus."

✝ I Peter 5:7—"Let him have all your worries and cares, for he is always thinking about you and watching everything that concerns you."

✝ John 14:18—"No, I will not abandon you or leave you as orphans in the storm—I will come to you."

✝ John 14:27—"I am leaving you with a gift—peace of mind and heart! And the peace I give isn't fragile like the peace the world gives. So don't be troubled or afraid."

- ✞ Psalm 46:1—"God is our refuge and strength, a tested help in times of trouble."
- ✞ Psalm 147:3-4—"He heals the brokenhearted, binding up their wounds."
- ✞ Isaiah 41:10—"Fear not, for I am with you. Do not be dismayed. I am your God. I will strengthen you; I will help you; I will uphold you with my victorious right hand."
- ✞ Roman 8:35-39—"Who then can ever keep Christ's love from us? When we have trouble or calamity, when we are hunted down or destroyed, is it because he doesn't love us anymore? And if we are hungry, or penniless, or in danger, or threatened with death, has God deserted us? No, for the Scriptures tell us that for his sake we must be ready to face death at every moment of the day—we are like sheep awaiting slaughter; but despite all this, overwhelming victory is ours through Christ who loved us enough to die for us. For I am convinced that nothing can ever separate us from his love. Death can't, and life can't. The angels won't, and all the powers of hell itself cannot keep God's love away. Our fears for today, our worries about tomorrow, or where we are—high above the sky, or in the deepest ocean—nothing will ever be able to separate us from the love of God demonstrated by our Lord Jesus Christ when he died for us." (All Scriptures are taken from the Living Bible Translation)

As you've just read some of the prescriptions that God has given for your healing, please read this story of how one woman depended on God to bring her out of a depressive episode in her life.

As the Spiritual Mother of the author of this book, I've witnessed how God has been a sustainer, encourager, healer, and deliverer in her life. Many days she wanted to give up completely, BUT BECAUSE God has given her a "mustard-seed grain of faith"—just enough faith to believe His Word—she was able to receive God's healing; YOU CAN TOO!! Even if you have not personally experienced depression, as you read this story, God can also use you to minister to someone else. Be Blessed and Receive God's Healing Word as you read this book.

Pastor Beverly L. Wilson

1st Lady of Valley Kingdom Ministries International

Foreword

Five years ago, I met this woman of God, Marilyn Okoye; there was a bundle of joy and energy in her, and it was delightful to be in her presence. To me, she was not a target for depression. But little do we know the road we have to travel in preparation for the gifts that are hidden in our spirit.

I knew there was something special about her. We, being of like spirits, were drawn together from that day to this. Her embracing smile and hearty laughter would always draw the good out of you. One could not be in a downtrodden spirit while she was in the room. The Shekinah Glory of God emanated from her. She became a daughter and dear friend to my family. I knew without a doubt that God had His Hands on this "Daughter of Zion."

As she embarked upon the journey of authorship, the paths that she took out of the pain and suffering became "Living Water Creations." In writing words of encouragement for others, even when it appeared to the natural eye that she should be totally overwhelmed and distraught, Marilyn inspired many as well as me. This is when God moved her to higher heights and deeper depths, thus "Overcoming Depression."

"Overcoming Depression, One Christian's Perspective" is written with a simplicity by which all can understand, be edified, and remain spiritually blessed. Marilyn has shown us that the words in Psalm 9:9-10 are true, and that's apparent in this book.

> *"The LORD also will be a refuge for the oppressed, a refuge in times of trouble . . . for thou, LORD, hast not forsaken them that seek thee"* (Psalm 9:9-10).

As you begin your journey of "Overcoming Depression" by reading this great book, open up your heart, mind, and spirit to receive the deliverance that is yours for the asking! I pray that as you read this book, you will be truly inspired to do as Marilyn did—**stand on God's Word of Deliverance!**

I am proud of you, Marilyn. May you continue to follow God as He directs your path.

Love,
Mildred L. Heath (aka Mom)

Introduction

When I've reached the end of my rope, in God's Presence, there's strength and hope.

When I've gotten to a place where I can no longer cope, in God's Presence, there's strength and hope.

When it seems my life is on a downward slope, in God's Presence, there's strength and hope.

For in His Presence, there is the anointing that destroys yokes, blessings without sorrow, counseling and deliverance, eternal life, faith, glory, healing, instruction, joy unspeakable, kindness and love, mercy, miracles, newness of life, ongoing forgiveness, patience, peace, power, preparation, protection, quietness in the midst of a storm, rest and restoration, salvation, songs, truth, understanding, virtue, vision, STRENGTH AND HOPE, for you and for me.

What a privilege it is to be in the Presence of God. Selah.

The place I knew I needed to be in order to overcome was in the presence of God. I knew that in His presence, I would receive my healing. Getting into God's presence is simply opening up the Bible and reading His word. It is praying to God. It is trusting God. It is allowing God to do what He wants to do in your life so that you will come out as pure gold, mature and equipped to do His will in your life.

My Perspective

My Perspective

In 2002, I had become depressed. I believe there were a number of factors that led to this depressive episode in my life. I was pregnant at age 35 with my third child; four months after the baby was born, my marriage failed; I became physically ill; my mom had taken ill; and, most importantly, I had not communicated with my heavenly Father as much as I should have. For some people, pregnant at age 35 with a third child is a joyous time, but I felt like I was starting over. Then I realized that God thought enough of me to choose me once again to bring one of His precious gifts into the world. Unfortunately, my husband and I had fallen out of agreement because of lies. The very foundation of the marriage had been severely damaged. I suffered from minor postpartum illnesses. My mom became ill and was plagued with other personal difficulties. Last but not least, I didn't pray and read my Bible like I should have. Now, I don't blame myself for all the things that happened, but I do believe that if I had been in direct communication with God, my heavenly Father, I would have been more able to handle the events that I faced. As the stress of my marriage increased, it became more difficult for me to get out of bed and go to work. Every morning, I would drudgingly get up and get the baby ready to go to the sitter.

After my husband would leave with the children, I would call in sick, get back in the bed and "cry myself a river." On the days I did make it to work, I would sit at my desk, unable to concentrate on the work I had to do. I only did enough work whereas I thought I would not get fired. To tell the truth, if it were not for the Lord on my side, I could have been terminated for any number of reasons. During all of this, I knew something was wrong, and I desperately needed help. I was not able to lean on my husband due to the breakdown in communication in our relationship. I was not able to lean on my mom due to the problems she was having in her life. I could not eat; I felt worse than sad. I could not focus. There were some days I could not get out of bed, and I began to have thoughts of suicide. Well, I had always been a joyous person, so

I purposed in my heart that this feeling of hopelessness and despair would not be victorious in my life. I Peter 5:8-10 says, "Be sober, be vigilant; because your adversary the devil, as a roaring lion, walketh about, seeking whom he may devour: Whom resist stedfast in the faith, knowing that the same afflictions are accomplished in your brethren that are in the world. But the God of all grace, who hath called us unto his eternal glory by Christ Jesus, after that ye have suffered a while, make you perfect, stablish, strengthen, settle you." Knowing that the Bible also says in Ephesians 6:13, "and having done all, to stand," I decided not to let depression overcome me without taking that stand. I sought the physical, mental, emotional, and spiritual help I needed to get my life back on track and in right relationship with God.

I'll never forget my first appointment in which I was assessed by a clinical therapist. The fact that I was seeing a male counselor only frustrated matters since all the hurt I had experienced in my marriage was so great. I did not want to say a word to him; I just sat there twiddling my thumbs. Moreover, I was uncomfortable with the fact that I was in the Psychiatric department. I started asking him questions like: "What are you going to do with the information I'm sharing with you? . . . Why do I have to see you first?" After he answered all my questions, he just sat there and waited for me to tell him what I thought was wrong. After talking with him, he suggested that I might be suffering from depression. I thought, "Yeah, right, I'm not depressed." From there I was assigned a therapist whom I met with once a week. Week after week I would talk about the hurt and betrayal I felt. She too suggested that I might be depressed. I started this book out by saying that I was depressed, but this was not an easy diagnosis for me to accept. After all, I was saved, and God was my Deliverer. My therapist recommended medication several times, but I declined. I told her that I believed God for complete healing.

After several weeks of declining medication, my therapist said to me, "Taking medicine for depression is like taking medicine for hypertension, diabetes, or heart disease, and we can credit God for the creation of these medicines." I still had some reservations and some fears. I felt if I took medicine for depression, I was not trusting God like I said I did. I felt embarrassed and ashamed to have to take this "kind" of medicine. I also felt that taking this medicine would not allow me to "function like normal." However, the day I could no longer get out of bed to get my 3-month-old baby ready to go to the sitter was the day I decided I would try this medicine. I had to do something; so I told the therapist that I would try the medication. I was put on a small dose of what is referred to as Selective Serotonin Reuptake Inhibitors (SSRIs). I must admit that even though my doctor said it could be 4-6 weeks before I would "feel better," I felt better in 4-6 hours. She said I was probably experiencing a placebo effect, but I believe it was a God effect! I give God all the glory because His ways are not our ways and His thoughts are not our thoughts (Is. 55:8—"For my thoughts are not your thoughts, neither are your ways my ways, saith the LORD"). What my doctor said could possibly take 4 to 6 weeks, God did in 4 to 6 hours.

The day after I started this medication, I was finally able to focus at work. Projects I had not done for weeks, I was able to finish within hours. All the thoughts that had been racing through my head finally stopped. I stopped crying as much and, praise God, even the thoughts of suicide had stopped. I do believe that as painful as this experience has been, God still has a plan for me. I believe God for complete healing and restoration of all things, and you can too. There are so many promises for us in the Bible. We just have to tap into God's truths. After having done all we know to do, we need to stand; for the battle is not ours—it is the Lord's (II Chr. 20:15—"And he said, Hearken ye, all Judah, and ye inhabitants of Jerusalem, and thou king Jehoshaphat, Thus saith the LORD unto you, Be not afraid nor dismayed by reason of this great multitude; for the battle is not yours, but God's"). I am so grateful to God that in the midst of it all, I understood that He was the key to my healing process, and in the midst of seeking help, my heavenly Father helped me, for He is a present help in the time of trouble (Ps. 46:1—"GOD IS our refuge and strength, a very present help in trouble").

Psalm 30:3

During this time, God had a blessing by the name of Mildred Heath, a true woman of God who prayed for me, counseled me, was a shoulder for me to cry on and who gave an ear to listen. One day, I had an appointment with my counselor and asked Mrs. Heath to watch my children. When I had come to pick them up, she was preparing to have Bible study. I asked if I could stay; she said, "Yes." She explained that what they usually did was read a passage of scripture and share with each other what God was saying to them from that verse. That evening, she had planned on reading Psalm 27, but her Bible was turned to Psalm 30. So she said, "Let's take turns reading Psalm 30." Psalm 30 has 12 verses. Verse three fell on me.

As I read, each word became alive to me, almost as if each one were jumping off the page: "*O LORD, thou hast brought up my soul from the grave: thou hast kept me alive, that I should not go down to the pit.*" The first thing I realized was that this was a point in David's life when he was depressed. As I pondered the fact that God had brought up David's soul from out of the grave, I knew right then and there that God would do the same for me. I knew that all the hurt and disappointment I had been experiencing would not end up becoming my grave, but God would bring me up and out. It goes on to say that God kept David alive; for me, God was saying, "You will live and not die (Ps. 118:17—"I shall not die, but live, and declare the works of the LORD"), and I will keep you alive." David professed that God would keep him alive and that he would not experience the emotional pit of depression.

When I read that, the Holy Spirit immediately revealed to me that the pit represented depression. I also understood that what God did for David, God would do for me. I want you to know that what God did for me, God will do for you. (Acts 10:34—"Then Peter opened his mouth, and said, Of a truth I perceive that God is no respecter of persons"). Psalm 30:3 gave me the hope, strength, courage, energy, wisdom, trust, and faith I needed to stand still and see the salvation of the Lord (Ex. 14:13—"And Moses said unto the people, Fear ye not, stand still, and see the salvation of the LORD, which he will show to you today"). Let me say that the stand was not easy. I still cried sometimes. Sometimes I wanted to do it myself; sometimes I didn't want to do it at all. Nevertheless, God had an appointed plan to draw me back to where I desired to be, and that was in direct communication with Him. Our Bible study continued for several weeks, and we were all encouraged by the Word of God. I encourage you to seek the Lord for yourself regardless of the season you may be experiencing, and let God be the "I Am that I Am" in your life (Ex. 3:14—"And God said unto Moses, I AM THAT I AM: and he said, Thus shalt thou say unto the children of Israel, I AM hath sent me unto you").

Depression

What Is Depression

I am not a doctor, therapist, or counselor; I am a child of the most High God. If you are experiencing difficulties in life—whatever they may be—I pray that you will be encouraged to try Jesus. Whether He heals you divinely or ministers to you through the aid of a professional therapist, it is God alone who gets all the glory. Depression is defined in many ways: feeling sadder than usual, feeling "down" longer than usual, feeling really "blue", not feeling like oneself, feeling hopeless, helpless, and worthless, or experiencing debilitating, emotional distress that lasts two weeks or longer. There has been no single cause related to the onset of depression. It can be the result of a combination of major events in one's life and, surprisingly, some of those events may not be "bad" or "negative" events.

Depression is also said to be linked to physical changes in the brain and connected to an imbalance of chemicals that carry signals to the brain and nerve cells called neurotransmitters. Some other factors that can lead to depression include: family history of depression, trauma and stress, death of a loved one, broken relationships, physical and/or other health conditions, a loved one's moving away, or a child's going off to college. Other psychological disorders could include: anxiety, eating disorders, and substance abuse.

Some physical causes of depression could include: onset of menstrual cycle and/or hormone deficiencies such as a fluctuation in the thyroid gland. Other symptoms of depression could include: difficulty concentrating, difficulty remembering, trouble sleeping, trouble making decisions, and loss of appetite.

What It Causes

Depression can cause you to lose pleasure in the things you enjoy. It can cause you to isolate yourself from family and friends. Depression can also affect your physical health with such illnesses as heart disease, stroke, cancer, diabetes and, ultimately, premature death. Depression can also affect and/or impair your ability to think clearly and make reasonable choices and decisions. You may think that your family members and friends are not concerned about what's happening to you. You may think that everyone has turned or will turn their back on you and that they are talking about the fact that you "are not quite yourself." You may think that everyone around you is thinking that you are mad at them or that you don't want to be bothered.

Again, you must understand that this is an illness that can impair your ability to reason or think clearly. Your family and friends may not know or understand how to approach you. They may be just as scared and concerned as you are about the changes in your mood and other areas of your life. Perhaps you may not be able to explain or understand what you are experiencing. Oftentimes, the negative stigma associated with depression leaves many people feeling too embarrassed or ashamed to discuss their situation or talk about it with anyone.

When someone suffers from diabetes or hypertension, he/she seeks the counsel of a medical professional, follows the instructions that are given, and takes any prescribed medications. Well, depression can be approached in the same way. If you are at the point of needing professional medical assistance, don't be ashamed to get the help you need.

What the Word says

In the Amplified Bible, Gen. 4:5 states, "But for Cain and his offering He had no respect or regard. So Cain was exceedingly angry and indignant, and he looked sad and depressed."

Cain was saddened because God did not receive his offering. Instead of repenting, Cain allowed his depression to impair his judgment, and he killed his brother.

The Amplified Bible also states in Luke 21:34, "But take heed to yourselves and be on your guard, lest your hearts be overburdened and depressed . . . ."

In this verse, if we are not careful of the choices we make and/ or not careful of the life we live, we can get caught up in a whirlwind of obstacles that can lead to depression.

In the Darby translation of Ps. 38:6, we find these words: "I am depressed; I am bowed down beyond measure; I go mourning all the day."

David had become depressed because of some of the foolish choices he had made and some of the things he had done.

Let's take a look at the life of Job. "After this opened Job his mouth, and cursed his day. And Job spake, and said, Let the day perish wherein I was born, and the night *in which* it was said, There is a man child conceived" (Job 3:1-3).

Job had lived an upright life before God, and there was no apparent wrongdoing on his part. Nevertheless, the afflictions in his life brought much distress and despair. Job had become depressed and cursed the day he was born.

Another noteworthy example is the life of Hannah. "Then said Elkanah her husband to her, Hannah, why weepest thou? and why eatest thou not? and why is thy heart grieved? . . ." (I Samuel 1:8).

> *Hannah had become depressed and downtrodden because she had not borne any children. During Biblical times, it was shameful to be without child.*

Our final example is found in the life of an ordinary woman. "And a certain woman, which had an issue of blood twelve years, And had suffered many things of many physicians, and had spent all that she had, and was nothing bettered, but rather grew worse, . . ." (Mark 5:25-26).

> *Imagine an illness of 12 years! She was considered an outcast. She had suffered this condition and exhausted all her resources with physicians, only to find out there was no help for her. Imagine her destitute and isolated life.*

What we see in the Word is that these people, faced with overwhelming difficulties in their lives, just as we are today, suffered from or experienced depression at some point in their lives.

Overcoming

Overcoming

Overcoming depression has been a daily walk that I do not do alone but, with the strength of Christ, I know that I am more than a conqueror (Rom. 8:37—"Nay, in all these things we are more than conquerors through him that loved us"). Two years ago, my life could have ended by way of my own hands; I had almost given in to the lies. Despite all the despair and hopelessness I was feeling, overcoming meant building myself up in the most holy faith (Jude 1:20—"But ye, beloved, building up yourselves on your most holy faith, praying in the Holy Ghost").

So, as I have stated before, I purposed in my heart that I would overcome. I cried out to God night and day. Sometimes I did not know what to say; it was during those times that I chose to simply believe the promises in God's Word. He promised that the Holy Spirit would make intercessions for me with groans that words could not express (Rom. 8:26—"Likewise the Spirit also helpeth our infirmities: for we know not what we should pray for as we ought: but the Spirit itself maketh intercession for us with groanings which cannot be uttered"); I received that promise by faith, and I truly felt the power of the Holy Spirit surround me with hope and love.

The Bible is filled with affirmations of victory concerning the trials of life, and I stand on them—not as a hearer only but as a doer also (Jas. 1:22—"But be ye doers of the word, and not hearers only, deceiving your own selves"). Revelation 12:11 says, "And they (the believers) overcame him (Satan) by the blood of (Jesus) the Lamb, and by the word of their testimony." So, as I tell this story of overcoming depression, I am telling my testimony as to how I purposed in my heart to overcome and how God awesomely delivered me from going down into the pit of depression.

Furthermore, it is my prayer that you would also purpose in your heart to overcome because greater is He that is in you than he that is in the world (I John. 4:4—"Ye are of God, little children, and have overcome them: because greater is he that is in you, than he that is in the world")!

Epilogue

The Bible says the devil is the father of all lies (Jn. 8:44—"...
When he speaketh a lie, he speaketh of his own: for he is a liar,
and the father of it"). If you don't already know and understand this, I
encourage you to read, meditate and seek revelation on II Corinthians
10:3-4 which says, "For though we walk in the flesh, we do not war after
the flesh: (For the weapons of our warfare are not carnal, but mighty
through God to the pulling down of strong holds;)," and Ephesians 6:12
which says, "For we wrestle not against flesh and blood, but against
principalities, against powers, against the rulers of the darkness of this
world, against spiritual wickedness in high places." In these verses, we see
our war is not against our sister or brother (a physical person), but it is
against principalities, powers, rulers of darkness, evils of this world that
we do not see, and spiritual wickedness in heavenly places. But, praise
God, we have mighty weapons of God that will pull down the stronghold
that depression could have in our lives.

I pray these next chapters of poems, prayers, and encouragements
shake the very foundation of anything in your life that has caused you
emotional, mental, and spiritual distress. I speak into your life that the
blessings of Isaiah 60:1-2 (AMP) are a constant reality in your life: "**Arise
[from depression and prostration in which circumstances have kept
you—rise to a new life!] Shine [be radiant with the glory of the LORD],
for your light has come, and the glory of the LORD has risen upon
you! For behold, darkness shall cover the earth, and dense darkness
[all] peoples, but the LORD shall arise upon you [O, Jerusalem], and
His glory shall be seen on you.**"

Jesus has already walked the earth healing every manner of sickness
and disease (Matt. 4:23—"And Jesus went about all Galilee, teaching in
their synagogues, and preaching the gospel of the kingdom, and healing
all manner of sickness and all manner of disease among the people"). We
know by His stripes we are healed (Is. 53:5—"But he was wounded for
our transgressions, he was bruised for our iniquities: the chastisement of

our peace was upon him; and with his stripes we are healed"). We read that over 2,000 years ago, men and women alike experienced depression; we also read that they trusted and believed, and the Word of God encouraged, healed, and delivered them. So, we can be assured that the emotional pit of depression did not escape the healing power of Jesus Christ; His power overcame it back then, and His power still overcomes it today, right now—right where you are!

For me, this was definitely a tough time, but I believe in my heart that it was not for me alone. Many wonderful things have been the result of what I had to endure. God birthed in me many wonderful poems and words of encouragement. My faith has increased. I gained wisdom, and I developed patience (something I had always asked God for). I am a better mother, daughter, sibling, friend and person because I chose to let God mold my character and not give in to the hurts and disappointments that I had experienced. The choice really is ours; it may not be easy, but it is not impossible because nothing is too hard for the LORD. (Jer. 32:17—"Ah Lord GOD! behold, thou hast made the heaven and the earth by thy great power and stretched out arm, and there is nothing too hard for thee").

Poems of Encouragement and Affirmations

A Letter from Your Dad

From the day I formed you in your mother's womb, I have been watching over you. Since before you were born and throughout all eternity, you must realize and understand you'll always be special to me. You have always been in my heart even though sometimes you feel miles apart. My child, I want you to know it is I who will bring you to an expected end; so, know now that the outcome is YOU WIN!! You are and will always be a part of my family, and I have reconciled you unto me to live righteously! You, my child, I have made an heir; I abide in you and will always be there. So, while you may feel miles away, close to my heart you'll always stay.

Sovereignly Yours,
God the Father

Jer. 29:11
Rom. 5:19
Titus 3:7
Col. 1:21-22
II Cor. 5:19-21 AMP

Made of You

Formed in my mother's womb, I knew not what I'd be, but You saw me and knew. Coming into this world, tiny, precious, trusting and thriving, I knew not what I'd be, but You looked at me and knew. Growing up with the entire world around me, I knew not what I'd be, but You called me and knew.

Accepting You in my life as my Lord and Savior, receiving You in my heart as my Healer and Deliverer, and knowing You as the Mighty God, the Everlasting Father and the Prince of Peace, I realized I'd be good and perfect and true because I now know that I am made of You.

Created in Your image, Your light shines in me. My life has been changed so that for Your glory, others may see. Strength and honor are mine; my mouth speaks Your wisdom, and my words are kind. Far more precious than rubies, I am abundantly blessed. I lie down in green pastures, and my soul finds its rest. Fearfully and wonderfully made, I am good and perfect and true. Created in Your image, I am made of You.

I Jn. 3:2
Prov. 31:10, 25-26
Jas. 1:17-18
Ps. 23:2
Ps. 139:14

I Will Live!

There came a point in my life when I wanted to die.
I wanted to die because of a lie.
This lie broke my heart. I almost fell apart.
I almost fell; I felt like hell had descended upon me,
Not knowing that the word "almost" would be the key.
You see, I said "almost" fell, but what really happened, I stand to tell.
I tell you it was God who lifted me from out of the pit
When my head hung low, my teeth I did grit.
You see, "almost" is not the end when to God your prayers you do send.
No longer depressed, no longer bound 'cause God has placed my feet on solid ground.
"Almost" fell? Oh, No! Not me! I stand to tell I live victoriously!
Hell, descend upon me? Oh, No! Not me! I stand to tell I walk in God's authority.
Me, die? Oh, No! Not yet! I stand to tell that I will neither let death nor life,
nor things present, nor things to come, nor any other creature separate me from
the love of God which is in Christ Jesus who has given me Life More Abundantly!

Rom. 8:38-39, Jn. 10:10, Ps. 30:3

Prayers of Encouragement and Affirmations

My Daily Prayer

*F*ather, I welcome You into this day; allow me to abide in You and You in me. May my footsteps be ordered and my words purposed, my thoughts captive and my actions focused on You. Let my will be submitted and Your Will Be Done.

In Jesus' Name, Amen.

"Abide in me, and I in you" (Jn. 15:4, KJV).

Unknown Feelings

Father, it is in Jesus' name that we come to petition Your throne of Grace to cover our needs and shortcomings. At times, we are overwhelmed with emotions and feelings we can't seem to control, but it is with good cheer that we know at all times You can comfort us if we just ask. So we ask You to comfort us. We ask for Your wisdom to guide us during these times of unknown feelings and to deliver us from any attack and trick the enemy is trying to place on us. We acknowledge You as Lord and Savior, the Lover of our souls, and we thank You for caring for us and allowing us to cast our cares upon You. We love You, and we adore You.

"Now unto him that is able to keep you from falling, and to present you faultless before the presence of his glory with exceeding joy, To the only wise God our Savior, be glory and majesty, dominion and power, both now and ever. Amen"

(Jude 1:24-25, KJV).

Scriptures of Encouragement and Affirmations

Remember to be aggressive because you are fighting for your life! The kingdom of heaven suffers violence, and the violent take it by force (Mat. 11:12). As you daily declare these words, take back your joy, peace, and hope by force!

1. I am an overcomer! (I John 5:4-5)
2. I am in Christ Jesus! (I Corinthians 1:30)
3. I am enriched in everything! (I Corinthians 1:5)
4. I am blameless! (I Corinthians 1:8)
5. I live in victory! (I Corinthians 15:57)
6. I am assured of reward! (I Corinthians 15:58)
7. I have the mind of Christ! (I Corinthians 2:16)
8. I am a temple! (I Corinthians 3:16)
9. I am a possessor of all things! (I Corinthians 3:21-23)
10. I am sanctified! (I Corinthians 6:11)
11. I am bought with a price! (I Corinthians 6:20)
12. I am walking in His light! (I John 1:7)
13. I am cleansed! (I John 1:7, 9)
14. I am anointed! (I John 2:20)
15. I am confident! (I John 4:17)
16. I have abundant life! (John 10:10)
17. I am confident of answers to prayer! (I John 5:14-15)
18. I am born of God! (I John 5:18)
19. I am courageous! (I Chronicles 28:20)
20. I am born again! (I Peter 1:23)
21. I have received mercy! (I Peter 2:10)
22. I am a newborn! (I Peter 2:2)
23. I am healed! (I Peter 2:24)
24. I am a living stone in a spiritual house! (I Peter 2:5)
25. I am built up! (I Peter 2:5)
26. I am a member of a royal priesthood! (I Peter 2:9)

27. I am chosen! (I Peter 2:9)
28. I am one of the people of God! (I Peter 2:9)
29. I am part of a new race! (I Peter 2:9)
30. I am being perfected! (I Peter 5:10)
31. I am called! (I Peter 5:10)
32. I am cared for! (I Peter 5:7)
33. I am changed! (I Samuel 10:6)
34. I have not been given a spirit of fear! (I Timothy 1:7)
35. I am standing firm in Christ! (II Corinthians 1:21)
36. I am given His Holy Spirit! (II Corinthians 1:22)
37. I am a warrior! (II Corinthians 10:4)
38. I am content in the midst of weakness! (II Corinthians 12:10)
39. I am controlled by the love of Christ! (II Corinthians 12:10)
40. I am made strong whenever I feel weak! (II Corinthians 12:10)
41. I am led in Christ's triumph! (II Corinthians 2:14)
42. I am triumphant! (II Corinthians 2:14)
43. I am the aroma of Christ! (II Corinthians 2:15)
44. I am transformed! (II Corinthians 3:18)
45. I am adequate! (II Corinthians 3:5)
46. I am a minister! (II Corinthians 3:6)
47. I am renewed! (II Corinthians 4:16)
48. I am a new creation! (II Corinthians 5:17)
49. I am a minister of reconciliation! (II Corinthians 5:18-19)
50. I am an ambassador for Christ! (II Corinthians 5:20)
51. I am rich! (II Corinthians 8:9)
52. I am abounding in grace! (II Corinthians 9:8)
53. I am given His magnificent promises! (II Peter 1:3-4)
54. I am glorified with Him! (II Thessalonians 2:14)
55. I am encouraged! (II Thessalonians 2:16-17)
56. I know in whom I believe! (II Timothy 1:12)
57. I am guarded by God! (II Timothy 1:12)
58. I am not ashamed! (II Timothy 1:12)
59. I am known! (II Timothy 2:19)
60. I am honoured! (II Timothy 2:21)
61. I am His soldier! (II Timothy 2:3-4)
62. I have understanding! (II Timothy 2:7)
63. I am equipped! (II Timothy 3:16-17)
64. I am His witness! (Acts 1:8)

65. I have power! (Acts 1:8)
66. I am justified! (Acts 13:39)
67. I am a light in a dark place! (Acts 13:47)
68. I am exalted at His right hand! (Acts 2:34-35)
69. I am filled! (Acts 2:4)
70. I am qualified! (Colossians 1:12)
71. I am rescued! (Colossians 1:13)
72. I am transferred into His Kingdom! (Colossians 1:13)
73. I am unblemished! (Colossians 1:22)
74. I am filled with the knowledge of His will! (Colossians 1:9)
75. I am complete in Christ! (Colossians 2:10)
76. I am circumcised spiritually! (Colossians 2:11)
77. I am on the winning side! (Colossians 2:15)
78. I am rooted and built-up in Him! (Colossians 2:7)
79. I am filled to the fullness of God! (Colossians 2:9-10)
80. I am hidden with Christ in God! (Colossians 3:3)
81. I am a fellow worker! (Colossians 4:11)
82. I am the head! (Deuteronomy 28:13)
83. I am established! (Deuteronomy 28:9)
84. I am secure! (Deuteronomy 33:12)
85. I am healthy! (Deuteronomy 7:15)
86. I have obtained an inheritance! (Ephesians 1:11)
87. I am predestined! (Ephesians 1:11)
88. I am included! (Ephesians 1:13)
89. I am marked! (Ephesians 1:13)
90. I am sealed by God with His Holy Spirit! (Ephesians 1:13)
91. I am guaranteed! (Ephesians 1:13-14)
92. I am enlightened! (Ephesians 1:18)
93. I am blessed! (Ephesians 1:3)
94. I am holy! (Ephesians 1:4)
95. I am adopted! (Ephesians 1:5)
96. I am accepted! (Ephesians 1:6)
97. I am forgiven! (Ephesians 1:7)
98. I am lavished with the riches of His grace! (Ephesians 1:7-8)
99. I am understood! (Ephesians 1:8)
100. I am created in Christ for good works! (Ephesians 2:10)
101. I am His handiwork! (Ephesians 2:10)
102. I am His workmanship! (Ephesians 2:10)

103. I am brought near! (Ephesians 2:13)
104. I am near to God! (Ephesians 2:13)
105. I have access! (Ephesians 2:18)
106. I am a fellow citizen with the saints! (Ephesians 2:19)
107. I am of God's household! (Ephesians 2:19)
108. I am alive! (Ephesians 2:4-5)
109. I am raised up with Christ! (Ephesians 2:6)
110. I am seated with Him! (Ephesians 2:6)
111. I am saved! (Ephesians 2:8)
112. I am strengthened in Him! (Ephesians 3:16)
113. I am a partaker of the promise in Christ! (Ephesians 3:6)
114. I am becoming a mature person! (Ephesians 4:13)
115. I am righteous! (Ephesians 4:22)
116. I am new! (Ephesians 4:24)
117. I am an imitator of God! (Ephesians 5:1)
118. I am cherished! (Ephesians 5:29)
119. I am a member of His body! (Ephesians 5:30)
120. I put on the whole armour of God! (Ephesians 6:11)
121. I am carried! (Exodus 19:4)
122. I am clean! (John 36:25; John 15:3)
123. I am crucified with Him! (Galatians 2:20)
124. I am redeemed! (Galatians 3:13)
125. I am clothed with Christ! (Galatians 3:27)
126. I am Abraham's offspring! (Galatians 3:29)
127. I am filled with the fruit of the Spirit! (Galatians 5:22-23)
128. I am created in His image! (Genesis 1:27)
129. I am the image of God! (Genesis 1:27)
130. I have received an unshakable Kingdom! (Hebrews 12:28)
131. I am disciplined! (Hebrews 12:5-11)
132. I am never forsaken! (Hebrews 13:5)
133. I am confident He will never leave! (Hebrews 13:5-6)
134. I am His sibling! (Hebrews 2:11)
135. I am a partaker of Christ! (Hebrews 3:14)
136. I am drawing near with confidence! (Hebrews 4:16)
137. I am a partaker of the Holy Spirit! (Hebrews 6:4)
138. I am betrothed! (Hosea 2:19-20)
139. I am heaven bound, guaranteed! (I Peter 1: 4)
140. I am obedient! (Isaiah 1:19)
141. I am stable! (Isaiah 33:6)

142. I am ransomed with Him! (Isaiah 35:10)
143. I am kept! (Isaiah 38:17)
144. I am delighted in! (Isaiah 42:1)
145. I am His! (Isaiah 43:1)
146. I am named! (Isaiah 43:1)
147. I am loved constantly, unconditionally! (Isaiah 43:4)
148. I am useful for His glory! (Isaiah 43:7)
149. I am helped by Him! (Isaiah 44:2)
150. I am unafraid! (Isaiah 44:2; 51:12)
151. I am the Lord's! (Isaiah 44:5)
152. I am refined! (Isaiah 48:10)
153. I am inscribed on His palms! (Isaiah 49:16)
154. I am rewarded by God! (Isaiah 49:4)
155. I am far from oppression! (Isaiah 54:14)
156. I am His bride! (Isaiah 54:5)
157. I am like a watered garden! (Isaiah 58:11)
158. I lack no wisdom! (James 1:5)
159. I am patient! (James 5:8)
160. I am formed in the womb by God! (Jeremiah 1:5)
161. I am clay in the potter's hand! (Jeremiah 18:6)
162. I am comforted! (Jeremiah 31:13)
163. I am satisfied! (Jeremiah 31:14)
164. I am pardoned! (Jeremiah 33:8)
165. I am favoured! (Job 10:12)
166. I am a child of God! (John 1:12)
167. I am abundant! (John 10:10)
168. I am indwelt by Christ Jesus! (John 14:20)
169. I am appointed by God! (John 15:16)
170. I am a branch of the True Vine! (John 15:5)
171. I am filled with joy! (John 17:13)
172. I am not of this world! (John 17:14)
173. I am sharing His glory! (John 17:22,24)
174. I am one with Him! (John 17:23-24)
175. I am God's gift to Christ! (John 17:24)
176. I belong to God! (John 17:9)
177. I am sent! (John 20:21)
178. I am loved! (John 3:16)
189. I have eternal life! (John 3:36)
180. I have passed from death to life! (John 5:24)

181. I am indestructible! (John 6:51)
182. I have life flowing through me! (John 7:38)
183. I have light! (John 8:12)
184. I am a disciple! (John 8:31-32)
185. I am set free! (John 8:31-32,36)
186. I am free! (John 8:36)
187. I am filled with might in God! (Luke 10:19)
188. I am welcome! (Luke 11:9)
189. I am valuable! (Luke 12:24)
190. I am watching for His return! (Luke 12:37)
191. I was lost, but now I am found! (Luke 19:10)
192. I have authority over the devil! (Luke 9:1)
193. I have power over the devil! (Luke 9:1)
194. I am a mountain mover! (Mark 11:22-23)
195. I am being made whole! (Mark 5:34)
196. I have rest provided! (Matthew 11:28-30)
197. I am yoked with Jesus! (Matthew 11:29)
198. I am the salt of the earth! (Matthew 5:13)
199. I am His representative! (Matthew 5:16)
200. I am provided for! (Matthew 6:33)
201. I have every good thing! (Philemon 6)
202. I am filled with the fruit of righteousness! (Philippians 1:11)
203. I am a finished product in progress! (Philippians 1:6)
204. I am confident He will finish me! (Philippians 1:6)
205. I am a partaker of grace! (Philippians 1:7)
206. I am empowered to obey! (Philippians 2:13)
207. I am a citizen of Heaven! (Philippians 3:20)
208. I have the power of God behind me! (Philippians 3:21)
209. I am content! (Philippians 4:11)
210. I am able! (Philippians 4:13)
211. I am determined! (Philippians 4:13)
212. I am amply supplied! (Philippians 4:18)
213. I am joyful! (Philippians 4:4)
214. I am anxious for nothing! (Philippians 4:6)
215. I am calm! (Philippians 4:6)
216. I am guarded by God's peace! (Philippians 4:7)
217. I have peace! (Philippians 4:7)
218. I am assured of success! (Proverbs 16:3)

219. I am wise! (Proverbs 2:6)
220. I am gracious! (Proverbs 22:11)
221. I am bold! (Proverbs 28:1)
222. I am prosperous! (Psalm 1:3)
223. I am made by Him! (Psalm 100:3)
224. I am delivered! (Psalm 107:6)
225. I am a bondservant! (Psalm 116:16)
226. I am purposeful! (Psalm 138:8)
227. I am thought about! (Psalm 139:17-18)
228. I am a delight! (Psalm 147:11)
229. I am beautiful! (Psalm 149:4)
230. I am pleasing to God! (Psalm 149:4)
231. I am His sheep! (Psalm 23:1)
232. I am a saint of God! (Psalm 34:9)
233. I am upheld! (Psalm 37:17)
234. I have my steps established by the Lord! (Psalm 37:23)
235. I am safe! (Psalm 4:8)
236. I am a King's kid! (Psalm 44:4)
237. I am desired! (Psalm 45:11)
238. I am guided! (Psalm 48:14)
239. I am in a wealthy place! (Psalm 66:12)
240. I am family! (Psalm 68:5)
241. I am a magnifier of God! (Psalm 69:30)
242. I am upright! (Psalm 7:10)
243. I am sustained from birth! (Psalm 71:6)
244. I am continually with God! (Psalm 73:23)
245. I am treasured! (Psalm 83:3)
246. I am loyal! (Psalm 86:2)
247. I am sheltered! (Psalm 91:1)
248. I am protected! (Psalm 91:14)
249. I am shielded! (Psalm 91:4)
250. I am His worshipper! (Psalm 95:6)
251. I am in a Kingdom of priests! (Revelation 1:6)
252. I am faithful! (Revelation 17:14)
253. I am worthy! (Revelation 3:4)
254. I am purchased! (Revelation 5:9)
255. I am a believer! (Romans 10:9)
256. I am gifted! (Romans 12:6)

257. I am abounding in hope! (Romans 15:4, 13)
258. I am reconciled to God! (Romans 5:10)
259. I am reigning with Him! (Romans 5:17)
260. I am granted grace in Christ Jesus! (Romans 5:17,20)
261. I am royalty! (Romans 5:17; 8:16-17)
262. I am standing in His grace! (Romans 5:2)
263. I am rejoicing! (Romans 5:2-3)
264. I am dead to sin! (Romans 6:11)
265. I am an instrument of righteousness! (Romans 6:13)
266. I am yielded to God! (Romans 6:13)
267. I am a slave to righteousness! (Romans 6:18)
268. I am liberated! (Romans 6:23)
269. I am buried with Christ! (Romans 6:4)
270. I am dead in Christ! (Romans 6:4)
271. I have new life! (Romans 6:4)
272. I am united with Christ! (Romans 6:5)
273. I am no longer a slave to sin! (Romans 6:6)
274. I am guiltless! (Romans 8:1)
275. I am not condemned! (Romans 8:1)
276. I am indwelt by His Spirit! (Romans 8:11)
277. I am a son of God! (Romans 8:14)
278. I am a co-heir with Christ! (Romans 8:17)
279. I am sharing Christ's inheritance! (Romans 8:17)
280. I am a first fruit! (Romans 8:23)
281. I know all things work together for good! (Romans 8:28)
282. I am becoming conformed to Christ! (Romans 8:29)
283. I know God is for me! (Romans 8:31)
284. I am freely given all things! (Romans 8:32)
285. I am inseparable from His love! (Romans 8:35)
286. I am a conqueror! (Romans 8:37)
287. I have life and peace in the Spirit! (Romans 8:6)
288. I am an object of mercy! (Romans 9:23)
289. I am prepared beforehand for glory! (Romans 9:23)
290. I am God's own possession! (Titus 2:14)
291. I am washed! (Titus 3:5)
292. I am an heir of God! (Titus 3:7)
293. I am the apple of His eye! (Zechariah 2:8)
294. I am humble! (Philippians 2:24)

Personal Affirmations

I Samuel 30:6

". . . but David encouraged himself in the LORD his God."

David and his army returned to their camp to find that it had been attacked and destroyed. Because the people were distraught over this devastation and had become angry with David, David had to encourage himself in the Lord. So it is at times with us when trials come and decisions have to be made. Get to a quiet place and begin to encourage yourself. Seek the peace and wisdom of God for your daily living.

Take some time and write out your own Affirmations

But whoever catches a glimpse of the revealed counsel of God—the free life!—even out of the corner of his eye, and sticks with it, is no distracted scatterbrain but a man or woman of action. That person will find delight and **affirmation** in the action (James 1:25, MSG).

God **affirms** us, making us a sure thing in Christ, putting his Yes within us (II Cor. 1:21, MSG).

_____

_____

_____

_____

_____

_____

_____

Listen intently to your heart and be encouraged in the Lord. Go **boldly** before the throne of Grace that you may obtain mercy and find grace to help in time of need (Heb. 4:16).

If God be for you, **no one** can be against you! (Rom. 8:31)

_____

_____

_____

_____

_____

_____

_____

_____

_____

_____

_____

_____

_____

_____

_____

_____

_____

_____

NOTES

NOTES